Chapter 1: Understanding Integrative Massage

Defining Integrative Massage

Integrative Massage is a therapeutic approach that transcends the boundaries of conventional massage therapy. At its core, it is a holistic practice that weaves together a variety of massage techniques and healing modalities to address the individual needs of each client. This method does not subscribe to a one-size-fits-all philosophy. Instead, it recognizes the uniqueness of every individual, tailoring the treatment to harmonize the physical, emotional, and energetic aspects of the person.

The origins of Integrative Massage are as diverse as its techniques, drawing inspiration from ancient healing traditions and modern therapeutic practices. It merges the wisdom of age-old therapies like Ayurveda Hot Stones and Traditional Thai Massage with contemporary approaches in bodywork. This fusion creates a rich, adaptable, and deeply effective form of therapy that is more than the sum of its parts.

Distinguishing Integrative Massage from Traditional Therapies

While traditional massage therapies like Swedish or Deep Tissue focus on specific techniques or areas of the body, Integrative Massage adopts a more comprehensive approach. It is not limited to just relieving muscle tension or promoting relaxation; it aims to create a holistic healing experience.

For instance, in a typical Swedish massage, the therapist might use long, flowing strokes primarily to relax the muscles and improve circulation. In contrast, an Integrative Massage session might combine these strokes with acupressure to target specific pain points, stretching techniques from Thai massage to improve flexibility, and even elements of energy work to balance the body's vital energy.

The Holistic Approach: Mind, Body, and Spirit

The true essence of Integrative Massage lies in its holistic approach. It acknowledges that physical ailments can be manifestations of imbalances not just in the body but also in the mind and spirit. Therefore, it aims to address the person as a whole.

- **Physical Wellness:** Through various massage techniques, Integrative Massage can relieve pain, improve circulation, and release muscle tension, contributing to better physical health and mobility.
- **Mental and Emotional Balance:** By creating a space of relaxation and mindfulness, Integrative Massage helps to reduce stress and anxiety. Techniques such as deep breathing and mindful awareness during the session can foster a sense of mental clarity and emotional calmness.
- **Spiritual Connection:** For many, Integrative Massage can be a deeply spiritual experience. The nurturing touch and the harmonious integration of different modalities can lead to a sense of connectedness and inner peace.

In summary, Integrative Massage is not just a therapeutic practice; it is a pathway to holistic health and well-being. By understanding its origins, distinguishing its methods from traditional massage therapies, and embracing its holistic approach, we can appreciate the depth and breadth of healing it offers. This chapter sets the stage for a deeper exploration into the benefits and applications of Integrative Massage, as we continue our journey through this eBook.

Hi Holistic Reader,

Welcome to a journey of healing and harmony. I'm Janet Carson, a licensed massage therapist and bodyworker specializing in the art and science of Integrative Massage. With years of experience and a deep passion for holistic wellness, I have crafted this guide to share the transformative power of combining various massage techniques.

I sincerely hope that this book proves to be a valuable companion on your journey toward wellness. My goal is to provide you with insights and techniques that will empower you to embrace a more holistic approach to your health. Whether you're seeking relief from physical discomfort, looking to enhance your athletic performance, or simply aiming to find a greater sense of balance and well-being in your life, the practices and philosophies discussed here are designed to help guide you every step of the way. May this book serve as a resource for nurturing both your body and mind, helping you to achieve a state of wellness that resonates deeply and positively impacts every aspect of your life.

With Warmest Regards,

Janet Carson

NCLMBT 16096

NPI 1578125084

The Holistic Path: Embracing Wellness Through Integrative Massage

Introduction

Welcome to a journey of discovery, healing, and holistic well-being. In this eBook, we explore the transformative world of Integrative Massage, a therapy that has been gaining remarkable momentum in the wellness community for its unique approach to health and healing.

At the heart of Integrative Massage lies a simple yet profound philosophy: the body, mind, and spirit are interconnected, and true wellness can only be achieved by addressing all these aspects in unison. This form of massage therapy stands out for its ability to blend various techniques, drawing from a rich tapestry of traditional and modern modalities. From the gentle, rhythmic strokes of Swedish massage to the targeted pressure of deep tissue work, from the energy-balancing practices of Reiki to the pinpoint precision of acupressure, Integrative Massage is a symphony of healing practices, tailored to meet the individual needs of each person.

As more people seek out holistic approaches to health, Integrative Massage has emerged as a frontrunner in this wellness revolution. It's not just a treatment; it's a journey towards a more balanced, healthy, and harmonious life. But with such a diverse array of techniques and approaches, it can be challenging to understand what Integrative Massage entails, how it can benefit you, and how often you should engage in this therapy for optimal results.

This eBook is designed to demystify these questions. Whether you're a seasoned enthusiast of massage therapy or a curious newcomer, my goal is to provide you with a comprehensive understanding of the benefits of Integrative Massage. We'll delve into how it can enhance your physical, emotional, and mental well-being, and guide you through determining the ideal frequency of sessions to suit your unique health and wellness objectives.

Join me as we unfold the layers of Integrative Massage, illuminating its potential to enrich your life, soothe your body, and uplift your spirit. Welcome to "The Holistic Path: Embracing Wellness Through Integrative Massage."

Chapter 2: The Benefits of Integrative Massage

Integrative Massage, with its comprehensive approach, offers a plethora of benefits that cater to the whole person — body, mind, and spirit. In this chapter, we delve into these benefits, understanding how Integrative Massage can be a key component in maintaining and enhancing overall health and wellness.

Physical Benefits

1. **Pain Relief:** One of the primary reasons individuals seek out massage therapy is for pain management. Integrative Massage effectively addresses this through techniques that target specific muscle groups, releasing tension and reducing pain. Whether it's a stiff neck, lower back pain, or muscle soreness, the varied techniques within Integrative Massage may offer relief.
2. **Improved Circulation:** The manipulation of soft tissues in massage therapy enhances blood flow. Improved circulation brings a wealth of benefits, including better oxygen and nutrient supply to the muscles and more efficient removal of toxins and waste products. This improved circulation can speed up recovery times and boost overall vitality.
3. **Enhanced Flexibility:** Regular Integrative Massage can increase flexibility and range of motion by loosening tight muscles and connective tissues. This is particularly beneficial for those with sedentary lifestyles or those who engage in physical activities and sports.
4. **Injury Prevention:** By improving muscle flexibility and circulation, Integrative Massage can also play a role in preventing injuries. Regular sessions can help identify and address any muscular imbalances or tensions that could potentially lead to injuries.

Mental and Emotional Benefits

1. **Stress Reduction:** Massage therapy is renowned for its ability to help reduce stress levels, and Integrative Massage takes this a step further. By combining massage techniques that are tailored for the individual Client's needs and possibly including energy and breathwork when appropriate, it promotes a deep state of relaxation, helping to alleviate stress and anxiety.
2. **Mental Clarity:** The relaxation and stress reduction achieved through Integrative Massage can lead to enhanced mental clarity and focus. Many clients report feeling more grounded and clear-headed after a session, which can improve productivity and overall mental performance.
3. **Emotional Balance:** The holistic nature of Integrative Massage acknowledges the connection between physical discomfort and emotional well-being. By addressing the physical aspects, it can also bring about emotional release and balance, leading to improved mood and emotional resilience.

Benefits for Chronic Conditions

Integrative Massage can be particularly beneficial for those suffering from chronic conditions. Here are a few examples:

1. **Arthritis:** Massage can help alleviate the pain and stiffness associated with arthritis, improving joint mobility and reducing discomfort.
2. **Migraines:** Regular massage sessions can reduce the frequency and intensity of migraines. Techniques that focus on the neck, shoulders, and head can be particularly effective.
3. **Fibromyalgia:** This condition, characterized by widespread pain and fatigue, can see significant benefits from Integrative Massage. It can help in managing pain, improving sleep quality, and reducing stress levels, which are often triggers for fibromyalgia flare-ups.

In conclusion, the benefits of Integrative Massage are far-reaching, addressing not only physical ailments but also enhancing mental and emotional well-being. For those with chronic conditions, it offers a complementary approach to manage and alleviate symptoms, contributing to an improved quality of life.

As we move to the next chapter, we will explore the various techniques that make Integrative Massage such a powerful and effective modality in the realm of therapeutic massage.

Chapter 3: Integrative Massage Techniques

Integrative Massage is a harmonious blend of diverse techniques, each contributing its unique healing properties to create a comprehensive and personalized therapy experience. This chapter will explore the various techniques employed in Integrative Massage and how these methods are synergistically combined for tailored client care.

Key Techniques in Integrative Massage

1. **Swedish Massage:** Known for its gentle, flowing strokes, Swedish massage is often foundational in Integrative Massage, promoting relaxation and enhancing circulation.
2. **Deep Tissue Massage:** This technique involves firm pressure and slow strokes to target deeper layers of muscle and fascia, addressing chronic pain and muscle tension.
3. **Reflexology:** Focusing on reflex points on the feet, hands, and ears, reflexology aims to stimulate various organs and body systems, promoting health and balance.
4. **Myofascial Release:** This technique uses gentle, sustained pressure on the myofascial connective tissue to eliminate pain and restore motion.
5. **Trigger Point Therapy:** It focuses on releasing tight muscle knots (trigger points) that can cause pain in other body parts.
6. **Medical Massage:** A targeted therapy aimed at treating specific medical conditions as diagnosed by a physician, often part of a broader rehabilitation program.
7. **Sports Massage:** Tailored for athletes, this technique focuses on the overused and stressed areas of the body from repetitive and often aggressive movements, aiding in injury prevention and recovery.
8. **Medi cupping:** This modern adaptation of cupping therapy uses vacuum therapy to create suction, lifting and separating soft tissues, increasing blood flow, and relieving inflammation.
9. **Passive Thai Stretching:** This involves gentle stretches and movements inspired by Thai massage techniques. It enhances

flexibility, improves range of motion, and helps release tension in the joints and muscles.

Combining Techniques for a Tailored Experience

In an integrative session, these techniques are not used in isolation but are woven together to address the client's specific needs. For example, a session might start with the relaxing strokes of Swedish massage, progress to deep tissue work for specific muscle tension, incorporate medi cupping for improved circulation, and conclude with passive Thai stretching for enhanced flexibility and joint mobility.

Case Studies: Examples of Treatment Plans

1. **Case Study 1: Office Worker with Chronic Neck and Shoulder Tension**
   - Treatment Plan: Begins with Swedish massage for relaxation, followed by trigger point therapy for specific muscle knots, and concludes with passive Thai stretching to improve neck and shoulder mobility.
2. **Case Study 2: Competitive Cyclist with Muscle Imbalances**
   - Treatment Plan: Combines sports massage for targeted muscle groups, deep tissue massage for tight areas, and Medi cupping for recovery, along with passive Thai stretching to maintain flexibility and balance muscle groups.
3. **Case Study 3: Senior Citizen with Limited Mobility**
   - Treatment Plan: Utilizes gentle myofascial release to address soft tissue restrictions, reflexology for overall well-being, and passive Thai stretching to gently enhance joint movement and flexibility.

These examples highlight the versatility of Integrative Massage, showcasing its capacity to cater to various needs, from general wellness and relaxation to addressing specific physical conditions or athletic performance requirements.

In the next chapter, we will explore the recommended frequency of Integrative Massage sessions to maximize health and wellness benefits.

Chapter 4: How Often Should You Get a Massage?

One of the most common questions in the realm of Integrative Massage Therapy is about the frequency of sessions. How often should one get a massage? The answer, like much of what pertains to Integrative Massage, is not one-size-fits-all. In this chapter, we will explore general guidelines for massage frequency based on different goals and needs and provide advice on determining the best massage schedule for you.

General Guidelines Based on Goals

1. **For Relaxation and General Wellness:**
   - **Frequency:** A monthly massage is typically sufficient for those seeking general relaxation and wellness maintenance. This regularity can help manage the everyday stress of life and work, keeping the body and mind in a balanced state.
2. **For Managing Chronic Pain:**
   - **Frequency:** For chronic conditions like back pain, arthritis, or fibromyalgia, a more frequent schedule may be beneficial. Initially, sessions might be scheduled weekly or bi-weekly to effectively address and manage pain. Once the condition is under control, the frequency can be reduced to a maintenance level.
3. **For Sports Performance and Injury Recovery:**
   - **Frequency:** Athletes or individuals recovering from injuries may benefit from more frequent massages, such as weekly sessions. This can help accelerate recovery, improve performance, and reduce the risk of future injuries.

Individual Needs and Conditions

1. **Acute vs. Chronic Conditions:**
   - Acute conditions, like a muscle strain from a recent injury, might require short-term, frequent massage therapy, such as twice a week until the issue is resolved.

- Chronic issues often benefit from a long-term, consistent approach, where the frequency can be gradually reduced as the condition improves.

2. **Stress Levels and Lifestyle Factors:**
   - Individuals with high-stress jobs or lifestyles might find greater benefits from more frequent sessions, such as every two weeks, to manage stress and its physical manifestations effectively.

Determining Your Best Massage Schedule

1. **Consult with a Professional:** A qualified massage therapist can assess your specific needs and help create a personalized massage plan. They can consider factors like your health history, current condition, and wellness goals.
2. **Listen to Your Body:** Pay attention to how your body responds after a massage. If you notice the benefits wearing off quickly, you might need sessions more frequently. Conversely, if you feel good for several weeks, a monthly schedule might be sufficient.
3. **Consider Your Lifestyle:** Your daily activities, stress levels, and time commitments play a significant role. Ensure your massage schedule aligns with your lifestyle and personal commitments.
4. **Be Flexible and Adaptive:** Be open to adjusting the frequency of your massages over time. As your body changes and responds to therapy, your needs may evolve.
5. **Budget Considerations:** Balance the ideal frequency with what is realistic for your budget. Even less frequent massages can offer significant benefits when part of a consistent wellness routine.

In conclusion, the frequency of Integrative Massage sessions should be tailored to your individual goals, needs, and lifestyle. It's a personal journey, and finding the right balance is key to maximizing the benefits of massage therapy.

In the next chapter, we will discuss how to maximize the benefits of your massage sessions and what complementary practices can enhance your Integrative Massage experience.

Chapter 5: Maximizing the Benefits of Your Massage Therapy

While the massage therapy session itself is crucial, what you do before, during, and after can significantly enhance its benefits. This chapter will provide you with practical tips to get the most out of your Integrative Massage sessions, suggest complementary practices that can amplify the effects, and discuss the importance of regular sessions as part of a comprehensive wellness routine.

Tips for Before, During, and After Massage Sessions

1. **Before Your Session:**
    - **Hydrate Well:** Drink plenty of water to hydrate your muscles for easier manipulation.
    - **Eat Lightly:** Have a light meal a few hours before the session to avoid discomfort while lying down.
    - **Arrive Early:** Arriving early can help you relax and mentally prepare for the session.
    - **Communicate:** Discuss your needs, concerns, and any areas of focus with your therapist.
2. **During Your Session:**
    - **Relax and Breathe:** Focus on breathing deeply and evenly to help relax your muscles and mind.
    - **Provide Feedback:** Don't hesitate to communicate if you need more or less pressure, or if something isn't feeling right.
    - **Let Go:** Try to let go of external thoughts and focus on the sensations and relaxation.
3. **After Your Session:**
    - **Hydrate Again:** Drink water post-session to help flush out any toxins released.
    - **Rest:** If possible, schedule some downtime after your massage to extend its relaxing effects.

- **Notice Your Body's Response:** Pay attention to how your body feels over the next few days.

Complementary Practices

Integrating other wellness practices can enhance the benefits of your Integrative Massage:

1. **Yoga:** Regular yoga practice can improve flexibility and strength, complementing the physical benefits of massage.
2. **Meditation:** Mindfulness or meditation can extend the mental clarity and stress relief gained from massage therapy.
3. **Hydration:** Keeping hydrated aids in muscle elasticity and overall health, supporting the work done during massage.
4. **Balanced Nutrition:** A well-balanced diet supports the body's natural healing processes, enhancing the effects of massage.
5. **Regular Exercise:** Gentle exercise, like walking or swimming, can maintain the mobility and muscle health encouraged by massage.

Importance of Regular Sessions and a Wellness Routine

1. **Consistency is Key:** Regular massage sessions can compound the benefits, particularly for chronic issues or stress management.
2. **Part of a Holistic Approach:** Consider massage as one component of a broader wellness plan that includes physical, mental, and emotional health practices.
3. **Adapt as Needed:** Be open to adjusting the frequency and type of massage as your needs and goals evolve.

In conclusion, to fully reap the benefits of Integrative Massage, it's essential to consider the entire experience - before, during, and after the sessions, alongside complementary wellness practices. Integrative Massage is most effective when it is a consistent part of a well-rounded approach to health and well-being.

In the next chapter, we will explore how to choose the right therapist and setting for your Integrative Massage, ensuring the best possible experience and outcomes.

Chapter 6: Choosing the Right Therapist and Setting

Selecting the right massage therapist and therapy center is crucial to your Integrative Massage experience. The effectiveness of your sessions can significantly depend on the skill, expertise, and environment provided by your therapist and their practice. This chapter offers guidance on what to consider when choosing a therapist, the importance of credentials and specialization, and how to ensure a comfortable and suitable environment for your needs.

Key Considerations in Selecting a Massage Therapist

1. **Credentials and Training:** Ensure your therapist is properly licensed and trained. Look for certifications from recognized institutions and ongoing professional development.
2. **Specialization:** Consider therapists who specialize in Integrative Massage or the specific techniques you require, such as sports massage or medical massage.
3. **Experience:** Experience can be a good indicator of proficiency. Inquire about their years of practice and areas of expertise.
4. **Communication Skills:** A good therapist should communicate effectively, listen to your needs, and be willing to adjust techniques accordingly.
5. **Client Reviews and References:** Client testimonials can offer insights into the therapist's style and effectiveness.

Choosing the Right Therapy Center

1. **Cleanliness and Hygiene:** The center should uphold high standards of cleanliness and hygiene, which is essential for your health and comfort.
2. **Ambiance:** The setting should be calming and conducive to relaxation, with elements like soft lighting, gentle music, and a quiet environment.

3. **Accessibility:** Consider the location and accessibility of the center, including convenience of scheduling and parking facilities.
4. **Privacy and Safety:** Ensure the center respects client privacy and follows safety protocols.

Checklist for Selecting a Massage Therapist

When meeting a potential therapist or visiting a therapy center, consider the following questions:

1. **What are your qualifications and certifications in massage therapy?**
2. **Do you have experience in Integrative Massage and its various techniques?**
3. **Can you provide client testimonials or references?**
4. **How do you tailor a massage session to individual client needs?**
5. **What is your approach to client communication and feedback during sessions?**
6. **Can you accommodate specific requests or health considerations (e.g., allergies, injuries)?**
7. **What measures do you take to ensure cleanliness and hygiene in your practice?**
8. **What is your policy on appointment cancellations or rescheduling?**

The relationship with your massage therapist is a personal and important one. It's crucial to choose someone who not only has the right skills and experience but also makes you feel comfortable and understood.

In the next chapter, we will discuss how Integrative Massage fits into your larger wellness journey, emphasizing its role in a holistic approach to health and well-being.

Chapter 7: Integrative Massage in Your Wellness Journey

Integrative Massage is not just a luxury or an occasional treat; it is a vital component of a holistic wellness strategy. This final chapter explores how Integrative Massage fits into the broader spectrum of health and well-being, offering practical advice on incorporating it into your overall health plan, and sharing inspiring testimonials from individuals who have experienced its transformative effects.

Integrative Massage as Part of Holistic Wellness

Integrative Massage should be viewed as a key element in a larger wellness framework, alongside other health practices. Its ability to address physical, mental, and emotional aspects makes it a powerful tool in maintaining and improving overall health. Integrating massage into your routine can help manage stress, improve physical function, and enhance mental clarity.

Incorporating Massage into Your Holistic Health Plan

1. **Regular Scheduling:** Incorporate regular massage sessions into your health regimen. Like exercise or healthy eating, make it a consistent part of your lifestyle.
2. **Combining Practices:** Pair massage with complementary practices like yoga, meditation, and balanced nutrition. The combination of these elements can amplify overall wellness.
3. **Listening to Your Body:** Use massage as a way to tune into your body's needs. It can help identify areas of tension or imbalance, guiding you in other aspects of your health and fitness.
4. **Stress Management:** Utilize massage as a regular tool for managing stress, which can have wide-ranging positive effects on your overall health, from improving sleep to boosting immunity.

Testimonials: The Transformative Power of Integrative Massage

1. **Case of Chronic Back Pain:**
   - *John's Story:* "After years of struggling with chronic back pain, Integrative Massage has been a revelation. Combining deep tissue work with stretching and relaxation techniques has given me relief I hadn't found in other treatments. It's now a non-negotiable part of my health routine."
2. **Overcoming Stress and Anxiety:**
   - *Emma's Experience:* "As someone who deals with high levels of stress and anxiety, Integrative Massage has been a game-changer. The sessions not only relax my body but also clear my mind. It's like hitting a reset button every time."
3. **Enhancing Athletic Performance:**
   - *Alex's Reflection:* "As an athlete, recovery is as important as training. Integrative Massage has become integral to my regimen. It helps in muscle recovery, prevents injuries, and I've seen a noticeable improvement in my performance."

These stories underscore the diverse and profound impact Integrative Massage can have. Whether it's managing chronic pain, combating stress, or enhancing physical performance, Integrative Massage offers benefits that extend well beyond the massage table.

As we conclude this eBook, remember that your wellness journey is unique, and Integrative Massage is a versatile and adaptable ally on this path. Embrace it as a regular part of your health and wellness strategy and experience the multitude of benefits it brings to your life.

Bonus Chapter: Harnessing the Power of Breath During Integrative Massage

Welcome to this special bonus chapter, dedicated to exploring the transformative role of breathing in enhancing your Integrative Massage experience. Often overlooked, the simple act of breathing can profoundly impact the effectiveness of your massage session. In this chapter, we delve into the art of breathing - a tool that is always at your disposal, yet holds untapped potential for deepening relaxation, releasing tension, and elevating your overall massage experience.

Introduction to the Power of Breath

Breathing is the bridge between the mind and the body, the subtle yet powerful conductor of our internal rhythm. During an Integrative Massage, synchronizing your breath with the therapist's movements can create a harmonious flow, allowing for a more profound release of tension and a deeper state of relaxation. By harnessing the power of breath, you engage actively in your healing process, turning a passive experience into an interactive journey of wellness.

In this chapter, we'll guide you through various breathing techniques that can be used before, during, and after your massage sessions. These techniques are designed to optimize your body's relaxation response, reduce anxiety, and enhance the therapeutic effects of the massage. Whether you're new to massage therapy or a seasoned enthusiast, mastering these breathing techniques can significantly amplify the benefits of your Integrative Massage sessions.

Join us as we explore the art of mindful breathing and unlock new dimensions of relaxation and healing in your Integrative Massage journey.

Chapter 8: Harnessing the Power of Breath During Integrative Massage

Breathing is more than a fundamental life process; it is a powerful tool that can enhance the therapeutic effects of Integrative Massage. This chapter delves into various breathing techniques that clients can use during massage sessions to deepen relaxation, reduce stress, and enhance the overall healing experience.

The Role of Breathing in Massage

Proper breathing during massage helps to relax the body, allowing muscles to release tension more effectively. It also aids in stress reduction and can enhance the emotional and spiritual benefits of the massage. By focusing on your breath, you engage more deeply with the process and create a meditative, restorative experience.

Breathing Techniques for Enhanced Relaxation

1. **Deep Diaphragmatic Breathing:**
   - *Technique:* Inhale slowly and deeply through your nose, allowing your abdomen to expand fully. Exhale slowly through your mouth or nose, feeling the abdomen contract.
   - *Benefits:* This breathing pattern activates the parasympathetic nervous system, promoting relaxation and stress relief.
2. **Rhythmic Breathing:**
   - *Technique:* Inhale for a count of four, hold for a count of four, exhale for a count of four, and then hold again for four seconds before repeating the cycle.
   - *Benefits:* Rhythmic breathing helps to focus the mind, reduces anxiety, and enhances the calming effects of the massage.
3. **Visualization Breathing:**
   - *Technique:* As you breathe, visualize a wave of relaxation flowing through your body. Inhale relaxation, and exhale tension and stress.

- *Benefits:* This technique aids in mental relaxation and can help in releasing emotional blockages.

4. **4-7-8 Breathing:**
    - *Technique:* Inhale quietly through your nose for four seconds, hold your breath for seven seconds, and exhale forcefully through your mouth for eight seconds.
    - *Benefits:* The 4-7-8 technique is known for its ability to quickly reduce anxiety and induce a state of calmness.
5. **Breath Focus Technique:**
    - *Technique:* Focus your attention on each breath without trying to change its pace or intensity. Simply be aware of your breath and let it flow naturally.
    - *Benefits:* This mindfulness approach to breathing helps increase awareness and presence during the massage.

Implementing Breathing Techniques in Your Massage Session

1. **Start with Breathing:** Begin your massage session with a few minutes of deep breathing to transition your mind and body into a state of relaxation.
2. **Communicate with Your Therapist:** Let your therapist know you are focusing on your breathing. They can help pace the session to your breath, enhancing the treatment's effectiveness.
3. **Use Breathing to Release Tension:** When your therapist is working on a particularly tense area, use deep, slow breaths to help relax the muscles and facilitate release.
4. **Post-Massage Breathing:** After the session, take a few minutes to continue deep breathing, helping to ground your experience and maintain the relaxed state.

By incorporating these breathing techniques into your Integrative Massage sessions, you can greatly enhance the therapeutic benefits, contributing to a deeper sense of relaxation and well-being.

Conclusion

As we reach the end of our journey through "The Holistic Path: Embracing Wellness Through Integrative Massage," let's reflect on the key insights and knowledge we've gathered. This eBook has been an exploration into the transformative world of Integrative Massage, a realm where various techniques harmonize to cater to the whole person — body, mind, and spirit.

Key Points Summary:

- **Understanding Integrative Massage:** We've delved into the essence of Integrative Massage, differentiating it from traditional massage therapies and highlighting its holistic approach.
- **Benefits of Integrative Massage:** The physical, mental, and emotional benefits of Integrative Massage, including its efficacy in managing chronic conditions, have been thoroughly explored.
- **Techniques:** A variety of techniques, including Swedish, deep tissue, acupressure, and specialized methods like medical massage, sports massage, and Medi cupping, have been discussed, emphasizing their synergistic effects.
- **Frequency of Sessions:** Guidelines for the frequency of sessions based on individual goals and needs have been provided, illustrating the importance of a personalized approach.
- **Maximizing Benefits:** Tips for enhancing the benefits of massage therapy before, during, and after sessions, and the integration of complementary practices like yoga and meditation, have been shared.
- **Choosing the Right Therapist:** The importance of selecting a qualified therapist and a suitable setting for massage therapy has been highlighted.
- **Integrative Massage in Your Wellness Journey:** We've emphasized the role of Integrative Massage in a holistic health plan, sharing inspiring testimonials to illustrate its transformative power.

Bonus Chapter - Chapter 8:

- **Harnessing the Power of Breath During Integrative Massage:** As a bonus, we explored how effective breathing techniques can augment the relaxation and healing process during Integrative Massage.

The Importance of Integrative Massage: Integrative Massage is not merely a physical therapy; it's a comprehensive approach to wellness. It stands as a testament to the power of combining various healing practices to address the entirety of an individual's well-being — physical, emotional, and spiritual. By embracing this holistic approach, you open yourself up to a world of wellness possibilities.

Should you wish to learn more, seek advice, or schedule a consultation, please feel free to contact me at:

Janet Carson

janet@indigoskymassage.art

www.indigoskymassage.art

I am here to support you on your path to holistic health and wellness. Thank you for joining me on this enlightening journey through the world of Integrative Massage. Here's to your health, well-being, and a balanced life.

Glossary of Terms

This glossary provides concise definitions of key terms related to Integrative Massage and its various techniques to help better understand the concepts discussed throughout this eBook.

1. Integrative Massage:

- A therapeutic approach that combines various massage techniques and modalities to address a wide range of physical, emotional, and spiritual needs.

2. Swedish Massage:

- A massage technique involving gentle, flowing strokes that promote relaxation and enhance circulation.

3. Deep Tissue Massage:

- A massage style that applies firm pressure and slow strokes to reach deeper layers of muscle and fascia, addressing chronic pain and muscle tension.

4. Acupressure:

- A traditional Chinese medicine technique that involves applying pressure to specific points on the body to alleviate pain and promote health.

5. Reflexology:

- A therapy that involves applying pressure to specific points on the feet, hands, and ears, believed to correspond to different body organs and systems.

6. Myofascial Release:

- A soft tissue therapy for the treatment of skeletal muscle immobility and pain, focusing on releasing muscular shortness and tightness.

7. Trigger Point Therapy:

- A bodywork technique that involves the application of pressure to tender muscle tissue in order to relieve pain and dysfunction in other parts of the body.

8. Medical Massage:

- A targeted massage approach that is specifically directed to resolve conditions diagnosed by a medical doctor.

9. Sports Massage:

- A form of massage involving the manipulation of soft tissue to benefit a person engaged in regular physical activity.

10. Medi cupping:

- A modern adaptation of the ancient art of cupping therapy, using vacuum therapy to create suction and promote healing.

11. Passive Thai Stretching:

- A technique involving gentle stretches and movements, inspired by Thai massage, to enhance flexibility and relieve muscle tension.

12. Holistic:

- Pertaining to the whole person, integrating the mind, body, and spirit in the quest for optimal health and wellness.

13. Fascia:

- A band or sheet of connective tissue, primarily collagen, beneath the skin that attaches, stabilizes, encloses, and separates muscles and other internal organs.

14. Chronic Condition:

- A long-developing syndrome or illness, such as arthritis or fibromyalgia, that often has complex causes and might not have a complete cure.

15. Acute Condition:

- A sudden onset of a disease or injury that is typically short in duration, often severe and rapidly progresses.

9 798321 620281